Meal plan for a Healthy body

Healthy muscles thanks to 40 fabulous quick and easy recipes that will help you lose weight and boost your metabolism.

Katia kolner

Test of Contents

Introduction

Vegan athletes need to be aware of what they eat and how much they eat to absorb the required nutrition that supports muscle function, repair, endurance, strength, and motivation as these are qualities that professional athletes' treasure. Protein features high on the list of what to eat. You should also consider your calorie intake, macro and micro nutritional sources and amino acids, some of which may need to be supplemented. Proteins and carbohydrates average at four calories per gram, while fats average at nine calories per gram. Following this, it is possible to calculate how much of each nutrient type to consume per day.

When planning your vegan diet, an athlete may need to consider their exercise routines, as those who gym may have high impact days (such as the dreaded "leg-day") and lower impact days where their bodies need more nutrients geared at repair work. For every athlete, their meal plans will be uniquely based on their age, weight, level of activity, food availability (veggies and fruits tend to be seasonal), and personal taste. You certainly don't have to eat buckets of beans to be a vegan.

Converting to the vegan diet from an omnivore diet may, surprisingly, be a huge mental shock; however, there are some changes to your digestive system to consider as well. Vegans consume more dietary fiber than most omnivores, hence, your gut may go through stages of feeling somewhat bloated. You will need to consume more water as well. There are many suggested ratios, yet the easiest is to work per calorie. A fast rule of 1 milliliter water per calorie seems easy enough to follow. Keeping in mind that the volume of your food may increase, you may also need to eat quite a while earlier than an omnivore would before exercising. So, the usual rule of an hour fast before eating may need to be extended to 90 minutes fast before exercising.

Always consider adding variety to your vegan diet as this increases the opportunity for your body to consume all of the vital amino acids, and this leads to better protein synthesis (which is essential for developing muscle tone and recovering from injuries). Plant-based meals are very filling due to their high fiber content, yet you need to consume a larger amount to meet your calorie requirements. To avoid feeling too sated, you can gain extra carbs from eating nuts and seeds throughout the day as snacks.

Finally, when adding the finishing touches to your training program, it is essential that you intersperse training sessions with sufficient time to ensure that your muscles have time to rest and recover (where you rebuild their energy reserves, hydrate your body, and restore the normal chemical balance of your metabolism). Short-term rest periods may be anything from taking a few minutes break before moving on to the next training activity or even taking the rest of the day off after a particularly strenuous session. Professional athletes know that the body may be a machine, but it is a machine that needs to have "down time" too. It would be best to do a training log where you record what you have eaten, how long you fasted before training, and how you felt during and after the training session. This will also help you to assess whether you need to add more carbs or proteins to your diet, and if you require a longer rest period before moving on to the next training activity.

If you struggle with fatigue (or the shakes) after strenuous activities, you may need to increase your amino acid consumption or get more zinc and iron into your system. Basically, we are all unique, and what works for another vegan athlete may not work for you. This training log can also allow you to experiment with perhaps moving to shorter training sessions with more frequent rest periods to achieve the same level of fitness and muscle building. No two professional athletes train the same way. Listen to your body and your gut to find a way that works for you.

Lastly, don't forget to get enough sleep. Mental fatigue can easily translate as physical symptoms. Insomnia may also be caused by a deficiency in magnesium. This could be caused by strenuous activity that consumes natural minerals in the body. Taking a magnesium supplement or eating some dark chocolate or half a banana before sleep can help create restful sleep.

Fortunately, the Internet allows for the development of support networks for vegan athletes. What we eat says a lot about us, and vegans can be successful, high-achieving athletes with planning and experimentation to find what works for their unique body.

Tips in Starting Plant-Based Diet Plan your Weight Loss

1. Make a list of 15-20 of your favorite foods

To make this list, sit down with your whole family and ask everyone about their favorite foods. Once this is done, look at the list and select those foods that are easy and quick to prepare and do not need too many ingredients.

The best if they are healthy meals.

2. Gather the recipes of the meals you are going to prepare

Organize your list. You can divide the meals into groups, for example: soups, meat dishes, vegetarian dishes and so on, so that it is easy to handle them.

Find the recipes you need and write them down or print them on sheets of paper. Also, you may consider buying a special notebook for recipes. The most important thing is to have easy access to them, because you will need them often.

3. Plan all-day meals

Don't just create a list of lunches. It is advisable to eat 3-5 times a day, so think about planning all breakfasts, lunches and dinners.

This will avoid eating out, it will help you plan and use your cooking time better. You will also have the opportunity to make better use of food leftovers (it is important if you want to maximize the savings effect).

4. Write your menu on paper

You have many ways to do it. You can use a notebook. On the other side you write a list of your meals, and on the right write all the necessary ingredients to prepare this meal (at one time you will have a meal plan and the shopping list).

Regardless of which method you choose, put your plan in a place clearly visible to all members of the house. The best place is the kitchen.

5. Check what you have in your pantry

Before putting your menu into action, it is a good idea to check your pantry, refrigerator and freezer first. Organize all the food you have there: throw away what is already expired, and order everything else in appropriate groups (go to the shopping list template to see an example of groups)

Plan meals based on the products you already have. For example, do you have pasta? Write pasta on your food list for the next day. If you like chicken pasta, but you don't have it, then write "chicken" on your shopping list.

In this way, you will reduce the supermarket account and also avoid unnecessary purchases of products that you already have at home. In addition, it is the first step to keep your refrigerator and pantry in order.

6. Adjust the menu according to your family's eventualities

When you are planning meals, consider your daily activities and those of your family. Did your children eat lunch at school? That day plan a more modest lunch at home. Do you come back late from work? Think of a dinner that takes little time to prepare. Has the family been invited to a Sunday dinner? You don't have to prepare dinner that day.

It is good to consider all the related factors and take them into account when creating your menu.

7. Use the seasonal products

Depending on the season, the availability of individual fruits and vegetables can change dramatically. Therefore, their prices also change. The best prices will be found during the harvest, which becomes savings.

The point is that it is normal that your menu can change during the year.

I recommend using fresh ingredients from your garden season or those that are available in the market this season.

8. Prepare more meals at once

Do you consider eating the same dish more than once in the week? Try to prepare a larger amount of this meal, for today and the next few days. If you do, put the food separately in containers and place them in the refrigerator or freezer, you can also bottle the food in jars.

Another example: for lunch you make chicken breast chops, and you also like salad with chicken breast. Cook more chicken breasts at a time and then store a part in the refrigerator. As a result, in the afternoon or the next day you will prepare your salad much faster.

9. Plan your food cleaning day

If ever by the end of the week you collect all the leftovers from your refrigerator, you can plan a night, when together with your family you will have dinner only leftovers.

That day you should also check which products are near the expiration date and these are the products to use in the meals of the next days. This way you reduce food waste and save money.

10. Review your daily plan

Your meal plan must be flexible. If necessary, don't be afraid to make modifications and use the opportunities.

Many people consider themselves choosy in food before switching to a plant-based diet. However, then they find food for themselves, which they could not even think of. Beans, tofu, different types of sweets from plants - such a meal for a meat lover seems tasteless. So, try a new dish and let your taste buds decide for themselves what they like best.

The 5 Determining Factors for Being Fit

It's is not easy to make a change in any diet that you quickly embrace. The decision to take on a plant-based meal plan is based on wanting to live healthier lives. The change might be inevitable later on after many realizations of what we get when we eventually abandon what we prefer to consume.

1. The first tip is all about setting rules and making sure that you are being initiated to new recipes of plant-based meals even twice a week. Regulations created by yourself will be quickly followed as compared to the ones formed and forced on you. In this plant-based diet, it is all about loving what you are doing. The created recipes will always be easy to follow, and once mastered, you will only be improving on them. One rule that can be created here is the setting of a day. This day is preserved mainly for one purpose, and that's making a plant-based meal. Make it to the family and get their ultimate reviews on what you have done. Ask them to comment on the tastes and the food in general. The result will help you a lot, especially in your next meal.

2. The next tip here is all about creating a constant tendency towards plant-based meals. Make a plan for cooking this food more often within a week. Don't wait for ages to pass

since you are getting induced to starting your plant-based diet. Practice makes perfect, and within a long time, your skills, especially necessary skills, will improve. Your experience will be a notch higher, and this will be reflected in your habits. Making cooking of plant meals frequent is one of the most excellent tips in jump-starting your plant-based meal. Along the way, you will get adapted to it. You'll also realize that you've changed your approach to how you always think of other types of food, such as diets full of meat and junk foods.

3. As a beginner in this diet, the best tip for starting a plant-based diet meal plan will be, to begin with, vegetables. Try your best to eat vegetables. The act can be during lunch and dinner or rather a supper. Ensure that your plate is always full of plants of different categories. Different colors can help you choose the different types you want to get to learn. Vegetables too can also be eaten as snacks, especially when combined with hummus or salsa. You can also use guacamole too in this combination and rest assured you will love it.

4. One tip that will help you in starting a plant-based diet meal is by using whole grains during breakfast. Use it in high quantities since it will help you in adopting this kind of diet within a short period. It is not always easy to use all of these whole grains. The best way forward is to choose meals that can suit you and the rest of your family at first. Good examples will be highly recommended. These might include oats, barley, or even buckwheat. Here, you can add some flavors provided by different types of nuts and several seeds. Don't forget to include fresh fruits next to your reach.

5. Another tip is about pairing foods. You can use this tool to have more excellent knowledge of which types of plant-

based foods can be matched and results in good taste. You can do this pairing by combining several flavors. The result should give you a strong feeling that works for you.

Appetizer and Snack Recipes

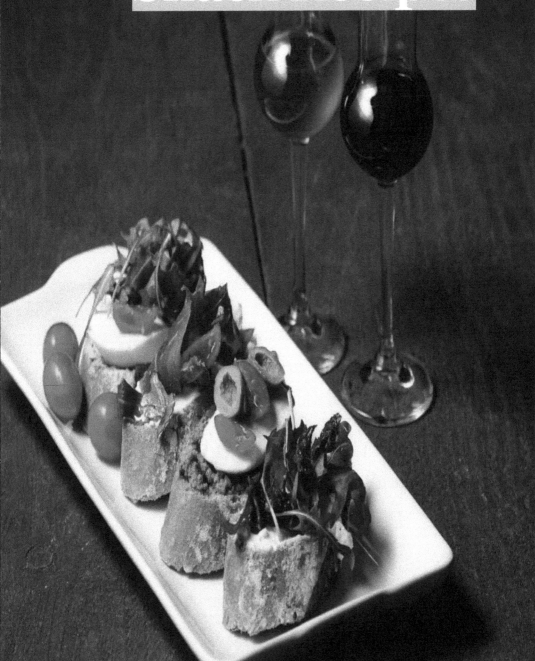

1. Acorn Squash with Mango Chutney

Preparation Time: 10 minutes

Cooking Time: 3 hours 10 minutes

Servings: 4

Ingredients:

- 1 large acorn squash
- ¼ cup mango chutney
- ¼ cup flaked coconut
- Salt and pepper as needed

Directions:

1. Chop squash into quarters and remove the seeds, discard the stringy pulp.
2. Spray your cooker with olive oil.
3. Transfer the squash to the slow cooker
4. Take a bowl and add coconut and chutney, mix well and divide the mixture into the center of the Squash.
5. Season well.
6. Close and cook on LOW for 2-3 hours.
7. Enjoy!

Nutrition:

226 Calories

6g Fat

24g Carbohydrates

2. Carrot Chips

Preparation Time: 9 minutes

Cooking Time: 11 minutes

Servings: 3

Ingredients:

- 3 cups carrots, sliced into paper-thin rounds
- 2 tablespoons olive oil
- 2 teaspoons ground cumin
- ½ teaspoon smoked paprika
- Pinch of salt

Directions:

1. Preheat your oven to 400 degrees Fahrenheit
2. Slice carrot into paper-thin shaped coins using a peeler
3. Toss with oil and spices
4. Layout the slices onto a parchment paper-lined baking sheet in a single layer
5. Sprinkle salt
6. Transfer to oven and bake for 8-10 minutes
7. Remove and serve
8. Enjoy!

Nutrition:

434 Calories4

35g Fat

32g Carbohydrates

3. Brussels and Pistachio

Preparation Time: 8 minutes

Cooking Time: 23 minutes

Servings: 5

Ingredients:

- 1-pound Brussels sprouts, tough bottom trimmed and halved lengthwise
- 4 shallots, peeled and quartered
- 1 tablespoon extra-virgin olive oil
- Sea salt
- Freshly ground black pepper
- ½ cup roasted pistachios, chopped
- Zest of ½ lemon
- Juice of ½ lemon

Directions:

1. Preheat your oven to 400 degrees Fahrenheit
2. In baking sheet and line, it with aluminum foil
3. Keep it on the side
4. Take a large bowl and add Brussels and shallots and dress them with olive oil
5. Season well and spread veggies onto a sheet

6. Bake for 15 minutes until slightly caramelized

7. Remove the oven and transfer to a serving bowl

8. Toss with lemon zest, lemon juice, and pistachios

9. Serve and enjoy!

Nutrition:

126 Calories

7g Fat

14g Carbohydrates

4. Buffalo Cashews

Preparation Time: 10 minutes

Cooking Time: 55 minutes

Servings: 4

Ingredients:

- 2 cups raw cashews
- ¾ cup red hot sauce
- 1/3 cup avocado oil
- ½ teaspoon garlic powder
- ¼ teaspoon turmeric

Directions:

1. Mix wet ingredients in a bowl and stir in seasoning
2. Add cashews to the bowl and mix
3. Soak cashews in hot sauce mix for 2-4 hours
4. Preheat your oven to 325 degrees Fahrenheit
5. Spread cashews onto a baking sheet
6. Bake for 35-55 minutes, turn every 10-15 minutes
7. Let them cool and serve!

Nutrition:

268 Calories

16g Fat

20g Carbohydrates

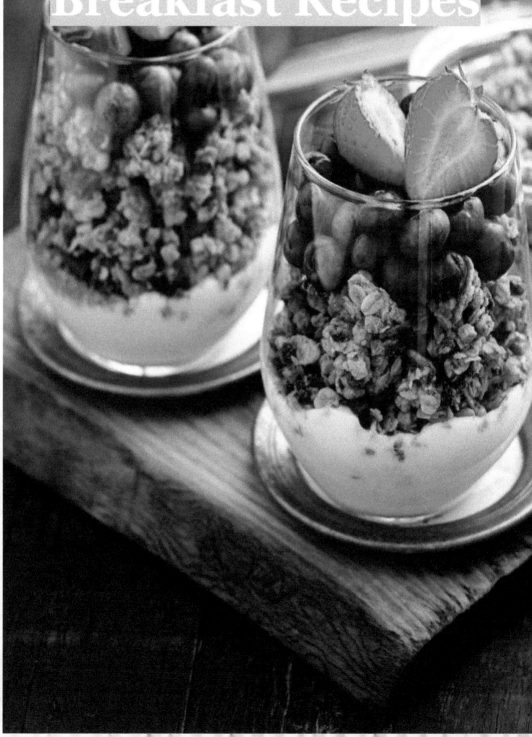

Breakfast Recipes

5. Pineapple Breeze Smoothie

Preparation Time: 5 minutes

Cooking Time: 0 minute

Serving: 1

Ingredients

- 1 (1-ounce) scoop vanilla protein powder
- 1 teaspoon-size piece fresh ginger
- 1 cup frozen spinach
- ½ cup pineapple chunks
- 1¼ cups unsweetened plant-based milk

Direction:

1. Blend all ingredients and process on high speed until smooth.

Nutrition:

148 Calories

2g Fat

22g Protein

6. Pumpkin Spice Smoothie

Preparation Time: 5 minutes

Cooking Time: 0 minute

Serving: 1

Ingredients:

- 1 (1-ounce) scoop vanilla protein powder

- ½ cup canned pumpkin purée

- 1 small frozen banana

- 1 teaspoon fresh ginger

- 1 teaspoon fresh turmeric

- ½ teaspoon cinnamon

- ¼ teaspoon nutmeg

- 2 tablespoons hemp hearts

- 1 teaspoon ground flaxseed

- 1¼ cups unsweetened plant-based milk

Direction:

1. Blend all ingredients and process on high speed until smooth.

Nutrition:

463 Calories

19g Fat

31g Protein

7. Mint Chocolate Smoothie

Preparation Time: 5 minutes

Cooking Time: 0 minute

Serving: 1

Ingredient:

- 1 (1-ounce) scoop chocolate protein powder
- ¼ cup fresh mint leaves
- 1 cup frozen spinach
- 1 small frozen banana
- 1 teaspoon spirulina
- 1¼ cups water

Direction:

1. Blend all ingredients and process on high speed until smooth.

Nutrition

253 Calories

5g Fat

24g Protein

8. Super Green Smoothie

Preparation Time: 5 minutes

Cooking Time: 0 minute

Serving: 1

Ingredient:

- 1 (1-ounce) scoop vanilla protein powder
- 1 cup frozen spinach
- ½ cucumber
- 2 celery stalks
- 1 teaspoon spirulina
- ½ small banana
- 1¼ cups water

Direction:

1. Blend all ingredients and process on high speed until smooth

Nutrition:

214 Calories

2g Fat

27g Protein

Main Dish Recipes

9. Curry Spiced Lentil Burgers

Preparation Time: 40 minutes
Cooking Time: 40 minutes
Serving: 6
Ingredient:

- cup lentils
- cups water
- carrots
- 1 small onion
- 3/4 cup whole grain flour
- spoons curry pow
- aspoon sea salt

mixture to stick. Form it into a ball. Scoop up ¼-cup portions.

4. Bake in baking sheet lined with parchment paper at 350°F for 40 minutes.

Nutrition:
114 Calories
1g fat
6g Protein

10. Maple Dijon Burgers

Preparation Time: 20 minutes

Cooking Time: 30 minutes

Serving: 6

Ingredient:

- 1 red bell pepper
- 1 (19-ounce) can chickpeas
- 1 cup ground almonds
- 2 teaspoons Dijon mustard
- 2 teaspoons maple syrup
- 1 garlic clove
- ½ lemon juice
- 1 teaspoon dried oregano
- ½ teaspoon dried sage
- 1 cup spinach
- 1½ cups rolled
- oats

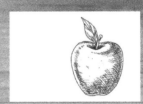

Direction:

1. Preheat the oven to 350°F. Line a baking sheet with parchment paper.

2. Chop red pepper in half, remove the stem and seeds, and roast on the baking sheet cut side up in the oven.

3. Crush chickpeas, almonds, mustard, maple syrup, garlic, lemon juice, oregano, sage, and spinach. Pulse until mix. When the red pepper is softened, blend along with the oats.

4. Scoop up ¼-cup portions and form into 12 patties, and lay them out on the baking sheet.

5. Bake for 30 minutes.

Nutrition:

Calories: 200;

Total fat: 11g;

Carbs: 21g;

Fiber: 6g;

Protein: 8g

11. Cajun Burgers

Preparation Time: 25 minutes

Cooking Time: 30 minutes

Serving: 3

Ingredient:

For dressing

- 1 tablespoon tahini
- 1 tablespoon apple cider vinegar
- 2 teaspoons Dijon mustard
- 2 tablespoons water
- 2 garlic cloves
- 1 teaspoon dried basil
- 1 teaspoon dried thyme
- ½ teaspoon dried oregano
- ½ teaspoon dried sage
- ½ teaspoon smoked paprika
- ¼ teaspoon cayenne pepper
- ¼ teaspoon sea salt

For burgers

- 2 cups water
- 1 cup kasha

- 2 carrots

- Handful fresh parsley

Direction:

For dressing

1. Whisk together the tahini, vinegar, and mustard until the mixture is very thick.

2. Stir in the rest of the ingredients. Set aside.

For burgers

1. Put the water, buckwheat, and sea salt in a medium pot. Boil for 2 minutes, then lower down heat, cover, and simmer for 15 minutes.

2. Once cooked, transfer it to a large bowl. Stir the grated carrot, fresh parsley, and all the dressing into the buckwheat. Scoop up ¼-cup portions and form into patties.

3. To bake them, put them on a baking sheet lined with parchment paper and bake at 350°F for about 30 minutes.

Nutrition:

124 Calories

2g fat

4g Protein

12. Grilled AHLT

Preparation Time: 5 minutes

Cooking Time: 10 minutes

Serving: 1

Ingredient:

- ¼ cup Classic Hummus

- 2 slices whole-grain bread

- ¼ avocado

- ½ cup lettuce

- ½ tomato, sliced

- 1 teaspoon olive oil

Direction

1. Lay out hummus on each slice of bread. Then layer the avocado, lettuce, and tomato on one slice, sprinkle with salt and pepper, and top with the other slice.

2. Preheat skillet to medium heat, and put ½ teaspoon of the olive oil just before putting the sandwich in the skillet. Cook for 3 to 5 minutes, then lift the sandwich with a spatula, drizzle the remaining ½ teaspoon olive oil into the skillet, and flip the sandwich to grill the other side for 3 to 5 minutes. Press it down with the spatula to seal the vegetables inside.

3. . Once done, remove from the skillet and slice in half to serve.

Nutrition:

322 Calories

11g Fiber

12g Protein

13. Black Bean Pizza

Preparation Time: 12 minutes

Cooking Time: 18 minutes

Serving: 6

Ingredient:

- 2 prebaked pizza crusts

- ½ cup Spicy Black Bean Dip

- 1 tomato

- 1 carrot

- 1 red onion

- 1 avocado

Direction:

1. Prep oven to 400°F.

2. Roll out two crusts out on a large baking sheet. Lay half the Spicy Black Bean Dip on each pizza crust. Then layer on the tomato slices and season.

3. Toss grated carrot with the sea salt and lightly rub. Arrange carrot on top of the tomato, then add the onion.

4. Bake for 15 minutes.

5. Top with sliced avocado and season.

Nutrition:

379 Calories

15g Fiber

13g Protein

Side Recipes

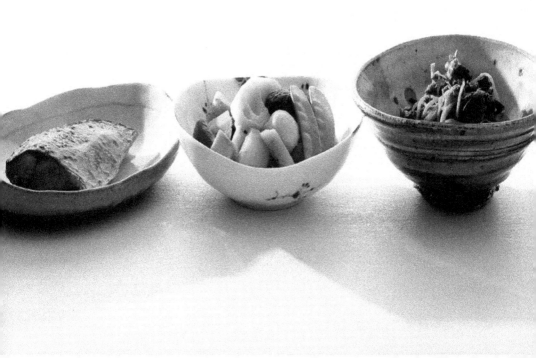

14. Aloo Gobi

Preparation Time: 15 minutes

Cooking Time: 5 hours

Serving: 4

Ingredients:

- 1 large cauliflower
- 1 large russet potato
- 1 medium yellow onion
- 1 cup canned diced tomatoes
- 1 cup frozen peas
- ¼ cup water
- 1 (2-inch) piece fresh ginger
- 1½ teaspoons garlic
- 1 jalapeño
- 1 tablespoon cumin seeds
- 1 tablespoon garam masala
- 1 teaspoon ground turmeric
- 1 heaping tablespoon fresh cilantro

Direction:

1. Combine the cauliflower, potato, onion, diced tomatoes, peas, water, ginger, garlic, jalapeño, cumin seeds, garam masala, and turmeric.

2. Cook low for 5 hours in slow cooker. Garnish with the cilantro, and serve.

Nutrition:

115 Calories

6g Protein

6g Fiber

15. Jackfruit Carnitas

Preparation Time: 15 minutes

Cooking Time: 8 hours

Serving: 4

Ingredients:

- 2 (20-ounce) cans jackfruit
- ¾ cup Very Easy Vegetable Broth
- 1 tablespoon ground cumin
- 1 tablespoon dried oregano
- 1½ teaspoons ground coriander
- 1 teaspoon minced garlic
- ½ teaspoon ground cinnamon
- 2 bay leaves

Direction:

1. Combine the jackfruit, vegetable broth, cumin, oregano, coriander, garlic, cinnamon, and bay leaves in a slow cooker. Stir to combine.

2. Cook on low for 8 hours. Shred jackfruit apart.

3. Remove the bay leaves. Serve with your favorite taco fixings.

Nutrition:

286 Calories

6g Protein

5g Fiber

16. Baked Beans

Preparation Time: 15 minutes

Cooking Time: 6 hours

Serving: 4

Ingredients:

- 2 (15-ounce) cans white beans
- 1 (15-ounce) can tomato sauce
- 1 medium yellow onion
- 1½ teaspoons garlic
- 3 tablespoons brown sugar
- 2 tablespoons molasses
- 1 tablespoon prepared yellow mustard
- 1 tablespoon chili powder
- 1 teaspoon soy sauce

Direction:

1. Mix beans, tomato sauce, onion, garlic, brown sugar, molasses, mustard, chili powder, and soy sauce into a slow cooker
2. Cook it on low for 6 hours. Season.

Nutrition:

468 Calories

25g Protein

20g Fiber

17. Brussels Sprouts Curry

Preparation Time: 15 minutes

Cooking Time: 8 hours

Serving: 4

Ingredients:

- ¾ pound Brussels sprouts
- 1 can full-fat coconut milk
- 1 cup Very Easy Vegetable Broth
- 1 medium onion
- 1 medium carrot
- 1 medium red or Yukon potato
- 1½ teaspoons garlic
- 1 (1-inch) piece fresh ginger
- 1 small serrano chili
- 2 tablespoons peanut butter
- 1 tablespoon rice vinegar
- 1 tablespoon cane sugar
- 1 tablespoon soy sauce
- 1 teaspoon curry powder
- 1 teaspoon ground turmeric

Direction

1. Mix Brussels sprouts, coconut milk, vegetable broth, onion, carrot, potato, garlic, ginger, serrano chili, peanut butter, vinegar, cane sugar, soy sauce, curry powder, and turmeric in a slow cooker.

2. Cook it low for 7 hours. Season. Serve

Nutrition:

404 Calories

10g Protein

8g Fiber

18. Jambalaya

Preparation Time: 15 minutes

Cooking Time: 8 hours

Serving: 4

Ingredients:

- 2 cups Very Easy Vegetable Broth
- 1 large yellow onion
- 1 green bell pepper
- 2 celery stalks, chopped
- 1½ teaspoons garlic
- 1 (15-ounce) can dark red kidney beans
- 1 (15-ounce) can black-eyed peas
- 1 (15-ounce) can diced tomatoes
- 2 tablespoons Cajun seasoning
- 2 teaspoons dried oregano
- 2 teaspoons dried parsley
- 1 teaspoon cayenne pepper
- 1 teaspoon smoked paprika
- ½ teaspoon dried thyme

Direction:

1. Mix vegetable broth, onion, bell pepper, celery, garlic, kidney beans, black-eyed peas, diced tomatoes, Cajun seasoning, oregano, parsley, cayenne pepper, smoked paprika, and dried thyme in a slow cooker.

2. Close and cook it low for 6 hours. Serve

Nutrition:

428 Calories

28g Protein

19g Fiber

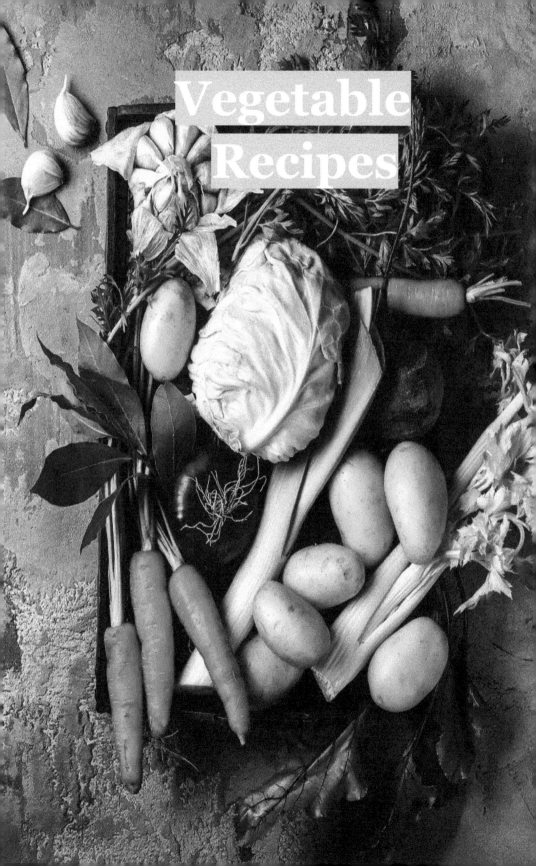

Vegetable
Recipes

19. Ratatouille

Preparation Time: 15 minutes

Cooking Time: 1 hour

Servings: 6

Ingredients:

- 8 baby eggplants
- 2 capsicums
- 4 medium tomatoes
- 4 zucchinis
- 2 onions
- 24–28 garlic cloves
- 4–6 tablespoons of fresh herbs
- Virgin olive oil for drizzling
- Salt and pepper to taste
- Balsamic vinegar

Direction:

1. Ready the oven to 400° and place a piece of wax baking paper on a large baking sheet.

2. If you're using baby eggplant, slice them in half lengthwise. Or, chop the full-size eggplant into roughly 1" bite-size pieces. Thickly slice the bell pepper / capsicum into inch-

wide strips, then cut in half. Cut the tomatoes into large chunks (roughly 6 chunks per tomato). Slice the zucchini the long way and then chop into ½ inch thick pieces. Likewise slice the onion in half, then into approximately half-inch thick half-moons.

3. Spread out the veggies on the baking sheet in a single layer, so none are piled up. Add the garlic gloves, not chopped – but do remember to peel them! Sprinkle the herbs atop.

4. Drizzle about ½ cup olive oil over the top and tilt the baking tray from side to side, ensuring the bottoms of all the veggies are well coated. The tops are still raw and not coated in oil, which gives them a lovely crisp texture when roasting.

5. Roast for 24 minutes, then flip the mix with a spatula and roast for another 10-15 minutes, or until the sides now facing up have been cooked visibly.

6. Turn down the heat to about 275-300°F and roast for another 15-20 minutes, or until the veggie mixture has become tender and the edges begin to caramelize (look golden brown, and taste sweet – you'll know that taste and smell!).

7. Season and serve immediately when hot. It serves very well with pasta, polenta, rice, in soft shell tortillas, or on a bed of fresh spring greens.

Nutrition:

147 Calories

2.5g Protein

9.7g Fat

20. Peanut Coconut Curry Veggies

Preparation Time: 13 minutes

Cooking Time: 27 minutes

Servings: 5

Ingredients:

- 2-5 tablespoons oil for frying

- 1 eggplant

- 1 zucchini

- 2 onions

- 2 garlic cloves

- 1-piece ginger

- 1 teaspoon cumin seeds

- 1 teaspoon of coriander seeds

- 1 teaspoon turmeric

- ½ teaspoon chili powder

- 1 can of coconut milk

- 1 tablespoon tamarind paste

- 1 tablespoon peanut butter

Direction:

1. Heat 1 tablespoon oil in a pan. Cook the eggplant / aubergine in batches until golden and soft, frying it for about 3-5 minutes per batch.

2. Take a medium-sized soup pot. Cut onion and add it to the pot with 1-2 tablespoons of oil and cook until soft and golden, somewhat translucent. Add the finely chopped garlic and ginger, and cook for a minute. Add the spices and cook for 2 more minutes.

3. Pour in the coconut milk, tamarind paste (or simply use fresh with a couple tablespoons of warm water) and peanut butter. Simmer gently for 2 minutes.

4. Add the cooked eggplant back into the pot and simmer for 15 minutes. Turn off the heat, stir through some finely chopped cilantro / coriander and serve with bread or rice.

Nutrition:

251 Calories

5.5g Protein

15.5g Fat

21. Stuffed Portobello Mushrooms with Walnut & Thyme

Preparation Time: 15 minutes

Cooking Time: 18 minutes

Servings: 2

Ingredients:

- 4 portobello mushrooms

- 4 tablespoons olive oil

- 1 yellow onion

- ¾ cup mushrooms

- 1 garlic clove

- 1 teaspoon smoked paprika

- 1 teaspoon thyme leaves

- 1 piece of day-old sourdough bread

- 2/3 cup walnuts

Direction:

1. Prep grill to medium. Cut the large stalks portobello mushrooms. Set aside. Rub portobello mushrooms with some frying oil on both sides, season, and grill for 6 minutes on high heat both sides.

2. Slice onion finely. Cut mushrooms, including the portobello stems, walnuts and toast. Crush garlic clove.

3. Get frying pan, set in medium heat, and sauté 2 tablespoons olive oil with the onion. Mix in the all chopped up mushrooms and a bit of salt. Sauté.

4. Stir pressed garlic, smoked paprika and thyme. Stir in the breadcrumbs and walnuts.

5. Scoop the mix into the middles of the portobello mushrooms. Grill again, for another 5 minutes.

6. Serve. Sprinkle nut cheese.

Nutrition:

306 Calories

11.4g Protein

18.8g Fat

22. Green Beans with Lemon Toasted Almonds

Preparation Time: 5 minutes

Cooking Time: 20 min.

Servings: 3

Ingredients:

- 1 pound of string beans
- ½ yellow onion
- 1 fresh lemon
- 1 ½ cup almonds
- 1 tablespoon Bragg's Amino Acids
- 3 tablespoons avocado oil

Direction:

1. After soaking the almonds overnight and letting them dehydrate / dry out, place them in a frying pan without oil on medium-low heat. Let toast for 5-8 minutes, stirring occasionally. Watch them carefully so they don't burn.

2. Meanwhile, trim the green beans and slice at a steep diagonal, into bite-sized pieces. Chop the onion.

3. Take a medium-sized frying pan, put in the oil and onion and beans. Sauté for 10 minutes, until the beans are al dente and the onion are translucent. Add the almonds, juice from the lemon (or ¼ cup lemon juice from a bottle),

Bragg's Amino Acids, and stir well, cooking for another 2 minutes.

4. Serve warm as a side dish, adding salt and pepper to taste.

Nutrition:

460 Calories

13.5g Protein

38g Fat

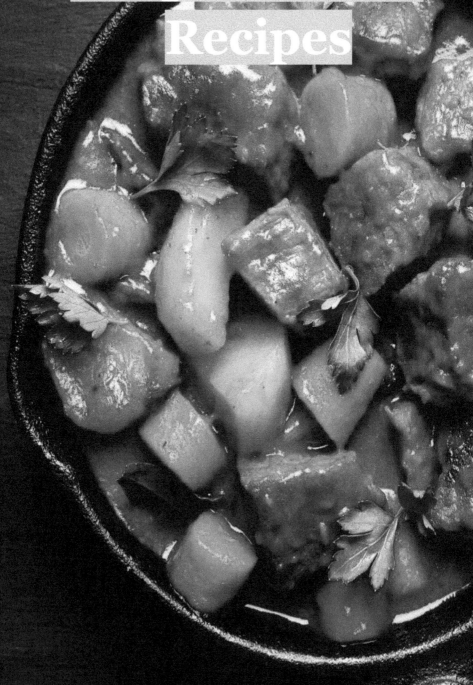

Soup and Stew Recipes

23. Tomato Gazpacho

Preparation Time: 30 minutes

Cooking Time: 55 minutes

Servings: 6

Ingredients:

- 2 Tablespoons Red Wine Vinegar

- ½ Teaspoon Pepper

- 1 Teaspoon Sea Salt

- 1 Avocado,

- ¼ Cup Basil, Fresh & Chopped

- 3 Tablespoons Olive Oil

- 1 Clove Garlic, crushed

- 1 Red Bell Pepper

- 1 Cucumber

- 2 ½ lbs. Large Tomatoes

Directions:

1. Place half of your cucumber, bell pepper, and ¼ cup of each tomato in a bowl, covering. Set it in the fried.

2. Puree your remaining tomatoes, cucumber and bell pepper with garlic, three tablespoons oil, two tablespoons of

vinegar, sea salt and black pepper into a blender, blending until smooth. Transfer it to a bowl, and chill for two hours.

3. Chop the avocado, adding it to your chopped vegetables, adding your remaining oil, vinegar, salt, pepper and basil.

4. Ladle your tomato puree mixture into bowls, and serve with chopped vegetables as a salad.

5. Interesting Facts:

6. Avocados themselves are ranked within the top five of the healthiest foods on the planet, so you know that the oil that is produced from them is too. It is loaded with healthy fats and essential fatty acids. Like race bran oil it is perfect to cook with as well! Bonus: Helps in the prevention of diabetes and lowers cholesterol levels.

Nutrition:

148 Calories

7g Protein

6g Fiber

24. Tomato Pumpkin Soup

Preparation Time: 25 minutes

Cooking Time: 25 minutes

Servings: 4

Ingredients:

- 2 cups pumpkin
- 1/2 cup tomato
- 1/2 cup onion
- 1 1/2 tsp. curry powder
- 1/2 tsp. paprika
- 2 cups vegetable stock
- 1 tsp. olive oil
- 1/2 tsp. garlic

Directions:

1. In a saucepan, add oil, garlic, and onion and sauté for 3 minutes over medium heat.
2. Add remaining ingredients into the saucepan and bring to boil.
3. Reduce heat and cover and simmer for 10 minutes.
4. Puree the soup with a blender.
5. Stir well and serve warm.

Nutrition:

180 Calories

10g Protein

5g Fiber

25. Cauliflower Spinach Soup

Preparation Time: 45 minutes

Cooking Time: 45 minutes

Servings: 5

Ingredients:

- 1/2 cup unsweetened coconut milk
- 5 oz. fresh spinach, chopped
- 5 watercress, chopped
- 8 cups vegetable stock
- 1 lb. cauliflower, chopped

Directions:

1. Add stock and cauliflower in a large saucepan and bring to boil over medium heat for 15 minutes.
2. Add spinach and watercress and cook for another 10 minutes.
3. Pull away from heat and blend the soup by using a blender.
4. Add coconut milk and stir well. Season with salt.
5. Stir well and serve hot.

Nutrition:

163 Calories

10g Protein

3g Fiber

26. Avocado Mint Soup

Preparation Time: 10 minutes

Cooking Time: 10 minutes

Servings: 2

Ingredients:

- 1 medium avocado
- 1 cup coconut milk
- 2 romaine lettuce leaves
- 20 fresh mint leaves
- 1 tbsp. fresh lime juice
- 1/8 tsp. salt

Direction:

1. Incorporate all ingredients into the blender until smooth. Soup should be thick not as a puree.

2. Pour into the serving bowls and place in the refrigerator for 10 minutes.

3. Stir well and serve chilled.

Nutrition:

187 Calories

11g Protein

9g Fiber

27. Creamy Squash Soup

Preparation Time: 35 minutes

Cooking Time: 35 minutes

Servings: 8

Ingredients:

- 3 cups butternut squash
- 1 ½ cups unsweetened coconut milk
- 1 tbsp. coconut oil
- 1 tsp. dried onion flakes
- 1 tbsp. curry powder
- 4 cups water
- 1 garlic clove
- 1 tsp. kosher salt

Directions:

1. Add squash, coconut oil, onion flakes, curry powder, water, garlic, and salt into a large saucepan. Bring to boil over high heat.

2. Select heat to medium and simmer for 20 minutes.

3. Puree the soup using a blender. Put soup back to the saucepan and stir in coconut milk and cook for 2 minutes.

4. Stir well and serve hot.

Nutrition:

180 Calories

9g Protein

7g Fiber

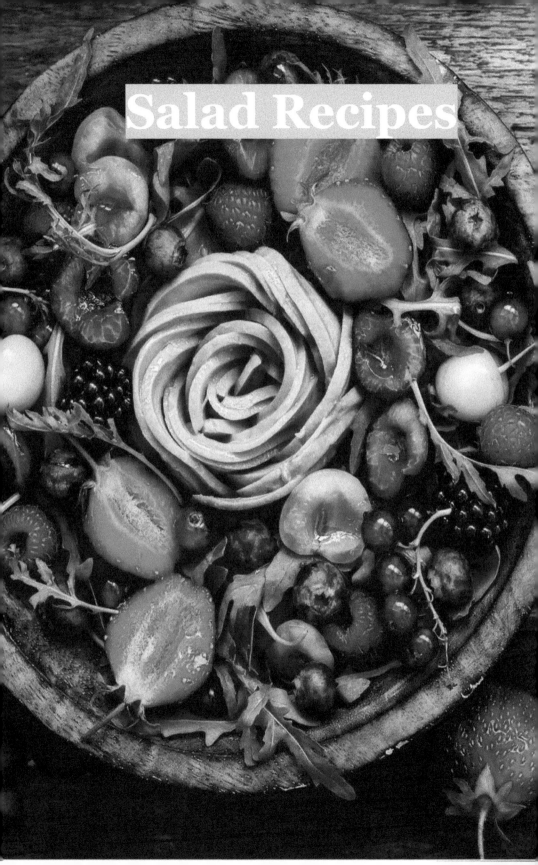

Salad Recipes

28. Ruby Grapefruit and Radicchio Salad

Preparation Time: 10 minutes

Cooking Time: 0 minute

Serving: 4

Ingredients:

For the salad

- 1 large ruby grapefruit
- 1 small head radicchio
- 2 cups green leaf lettuce
- 2 cups baby spinach
- 1 bunch watercress
- 6 radishes, sliced paper-thin

For the dressing

- Juice of 1 lemon
- 2 teaspoons agave
- 1 teaspoon white wine vinegar
- ½ teaspoon sea salt
- ½ teaspoon black pepper
- ¼ cup olive oil

Direction:

For salad:

1. Cut both ends off of the grapefruit, stand it on a cutting board on one of the flat sides, and, using a sharp knife, cut away the peel and all of the white pith. Remove the individual segments by slicing between the membrane and fruit on each side of each segment, dropping the fruit into a large salad bowl as you go.

2. Add the radicchio, lettuce, spinach, watercress, and radishes to the bowl and toss well.

For dressing:

3. Whisk together the lemon juice, agave, vinegar, salt, and pepper. Slowly whisk in the olive oil and mix.

4. Toss the salad with the dressing.

Nutrition:

148 Calories

5g Protein

4g Fiber

29. Apple and Ginger Slaw

Preparation Time: 10 minutes

Cooking Time: 0 minute

Serving: 4

Ingredients:

- 2 tablespoons olive oil
- 1 lemon juice
- 1 teaspoon ginger
- 2 apples
- 4 cups red cabbage

Direction:

1. Scourge olive oil, lemon juice, ginger, and salt and set aside.
2. Mix the apples and cabbage. Toss with the vinaigrette and serve immediately.

Nutrition:

190 Calories

10g Protein

4g Fiber

30. Spinach and Pomegranate Salad

Preparation Time: 10 minutes

Cooking Time: 0 minute

Serving: 4

Ingredient:

- 10 ounces baby spinach
- 1 pomegranate's seed
- 1 cup fresh blackberries
- ¼ red onion
- ½ cup pecans
- ¼ cup balsamic vinegar
- ¾ cup olive oil
- ½ teaspoon salt
- ½ teaspoon black pepper

Direction

1. Mix spinach, pomegranate seeds, blackberries, red onion, and pecans.

2. Scourge together the vinegar, olive oil, salt, and pepper. Toss with the salad and serve immediately.

Nutrition:

218 Calories

9g Protein

6g Fiber

31. Pear Veggie Salad

Preparation Time: 13 minutes

Cooking Time: 8 minutes

Serving: 3

Ingredient:

- ¼ Cup pecans
- 10 ounces arugula
- 2 pears
- 1 tablespoon shallot
- 2 tablespoons champagne vinegar
- 2 tablespoons olive oil
- ¼ teaspoon salt
- ¼ teaspoon black pepper
- ¼ teaspoon Dijon mustard

Direction:

1. Preheat the oven to 350°F. Arrange pecans in 1 layer on a baking sheet. Toast in the preheated oven until fragrant, about 6 minutes. Remove from the oven and let cool.

2. Toss the pecans, arugula, and pears.

3. Scourge together the shallot, vinegar, olive oil, salt, pepper, and -mustard. Toss with the salad and serve immediately.

Nutrition:

198 Calories

10g Protein

2g Fiber

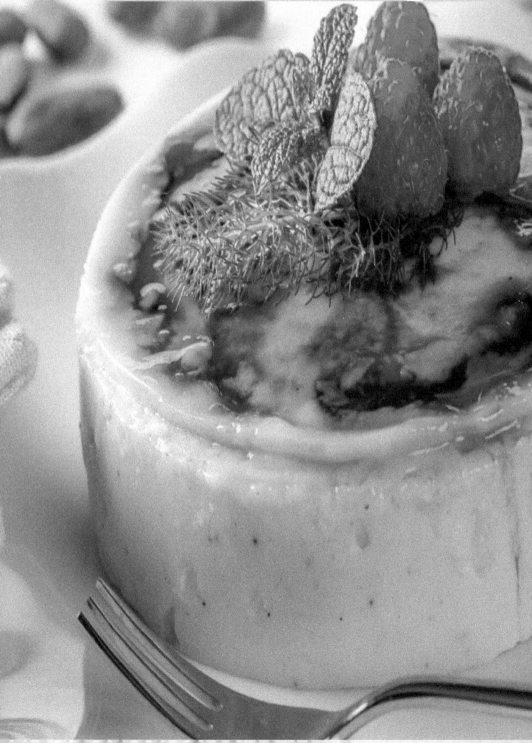

32. Banana Chocolate Cupcakes

Preparation Time: 20 minutes

Cooking Time: 20 minutes

Servings: 12

Ingredients

- 3 medium bananas
- 1 cup non-dairy milk
- 2 tablespoons almond butter
- 1 teaspoon apple cider vinegar
- 1 teaspoon pure vanilla extract
- 1¼ cups whole-grain flour
- ½ Cup rolled oats
- ¼ Cup coconut sugar (optional)
- 1 teaspoon baking powder
- ½ Teaspoon baking soda
- ½ Cup unsweetened cocoa powder
- ¼ Cup chia seeds, or sesame seeds
- ¼ Cup dark chocolate chips, dried cranberries, or raisins (optional)

Directions:

1. Preheat the oven to 350°f. Lightly grease the cups of two 6-cup muffin tins.

2. Put the bananas, milk, almond butter, vinegar, and vanilla in a blender and purée until smooth.

3. Put the flour, oats, sugar (if using), baking powder, baking soda, cocoa powder, chia seeds, salt, and chocolate chips in another large bowl, and stir to combine. Mix together the wet and dry Ingredients, stirring as little as possible. Portion into muffin cups, and bake for 20 to 25 minutes.

Nutrition

215 calories

9g fiber

6g protein

33. Minty Fruit Salad

Preparation Time: 15 minutes

Cooking Time: 5 minutes

Servings: 4

Ingredients

- ¼ Cup lemon juice

- 4 teaspoons maple syrup

- 2 cups chopped pineapple

- 2 cups chopped strawberries

- 2 cups raspberries

- 1 cup blueberries

- 8 fresh mint leaves

Directions:

1. Incorporate Ingredients in this order:

2. A tbsp. of lemon juice, 1 tsp. of maple syrup, ½ cup of pineapple, ½ cup of strawberries, ½ cup of raspberries, ¼ cup of blueberries, and 2 mint leaves.

3. Repeat to fill 3 more jars. Close the jars tightly with lids.

Nutrition:

138 calories

1g fat

2g protein

34. Mango Coconut Cream Pie

Preparation time: 50 minutes

Cooking Time: 0 minute

Servings: 8

Ingredients

For crust

- ½ Cup rolled oats

- 1 cup cashews

- 1 cup soft pitted dates

For filling

- 1 cup canned coconut milk

- ½ Cup water

- 2 large mangos

- ½ Cup unsweetened shredded coconut

Directions:

1. Situate all the crust Ingredients in a food processor and pulse until it holds together. Press the mixture down firmly into an 8-inch pie or spring form pan.

2. Put the all filling Ingredients in a blender and purée until smooth (about 1 minute).

3. Position filling into the crust, use a rubber spatula to smooth the top, and freeze for 30 minutes. Once frozen, it should be set out for about 15 minutes to soften before serving.

4. Top with a batch of coconut whipped cream scooped on top of the pie once it's set. Topped off with a sprinkling of toasted shredded coconut.

Nutrition

427 calories

28g total fat

8g protein

35. Cherry-Vanilla Rice Pudding

Preparation Time: 5 minutes

Cooking Time: 0 minute

Serving: 6

Ingredients

- 1 cup short-grain brown rice
- 1¾ cups nondairy milk
- 1½ cups water
- 4 tablespoons pure maple syrup
- 1 teaspoon vanilla extract
- Pinch salt
- ¼ Cup dried cherries

Directions

1. In your electric pressure cooker's cooking pot, combine the rice, milk, water, sugar, vanilla, and salt.

2. High pressure for 30 minutes. Seal, and select high pressure for 30 minutes.

3. Pressure release. Once complete, allow pressure release naturally, about 20 minutes. Unlock and remove the lid. Stir in the cherries and put the lid back on loosely for about 10 minutes. Serve, adding more milk or sugar, as desired.

Nutrition

177 calories

3g protein

2g fiber

36. Mint Chocolate Chip Sorbet

Preparation Time: 5 minutes

Cooking Time: 0 minute

Servings: 1

Ingredients

- 1 frozen banana

- 1 tablespoon almond butter

- 2 tablespoons fresh mint

- ¼ Cup or less non-dairy milk

- 3 tablespoons non-dairy chocolate chips

- 3 tablespoons goji berries

Directions:

1. Put the banana, almond butter, and mint in a food processor or blender and purée until smooth.

2. Add the non-dairy milk if needed to keep blending. Pulse the chocolate chips and goji berries (if using) into the mix so they're roughly chopped up.

Nutrition

212 calories

4g fiber

3g protein

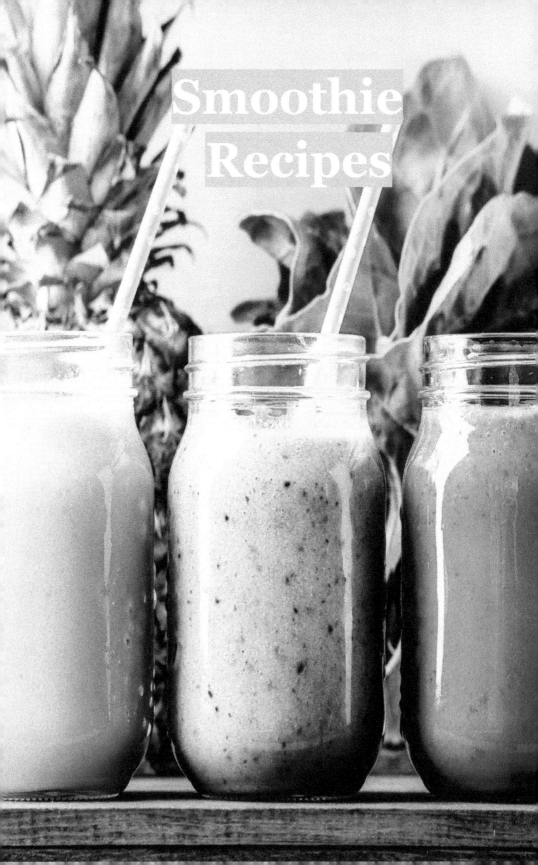

Smoothie
Recipes

37. Healthy Green Smoothie

Preparation Time: 10 minutes

Cooking Time: 0 minute

Serving: 2

Ingredients:

- 2 cups baby spinach leaves
- 1 stalk celery
- 1 cucumber
- 1 cup water

Directions:

1.   Place the spinach, celery and cucumber in a high-speed blender and blend until smooth.

2.   Add the water or ice and blend.

Nutrition

200 Calories

1.7g Fiber

2g Protein

38.   Chocolate Mint Smoothie

Preparation Time: 15 minutes

Cooking Time: 0 minute

Serving: 2

Ingredients:

- ¾ cup plain Greek Yogurt

- 1 cup almond milk

- ¼ cup fresh mint

- 1 cup baby spinach leaves

- 1 tablespoon maple syrup

- ¼ cup semi-sweet chocolate chips

- 2 cups ice

Directions:

1.   Place the yogurt, milk, mint and spinach in a blender and blend on high until frothy.

2.   Add the maple syrup and chocolate chips and blend a few seconds to break up the chocolate chips.

3.   Add the ice and blend until thick and smooth.

Nutrition

170 Calories

5g Fiber

8g Protein

39. Coco Milk Smoothie

Preparation Time: 4 minutes

Cooking Time: 2 minutes

Servings: 1

Ingredients:

- 1 t. chia seeds

- 1/8 c. almonds

- 1 c. coconut milk

- 1 avocado

Directions:

1. Incorporate all the ingredients.
2. Stir in desired number of ice cubes then blend again.

Nutrition:

584 Calories

22.5g Carbohydrates

8.3g Proteins

40. Almond Smoothie

Preparation Time: 6 minutes

Cooking Time: 4 minutes

Servings: 3

Ingredients:

- ½ tsp. vanilla extract

- 1 scoop maca powder

- 1 tbsp. almond butter

- 1 cup almond milk, unsweetened

- 2 avocados

Directions:

1. Blend all the ingredients until smooth.

Nutrition:

758 Calories

28g Carbohydrates

9g Proteins

30-Day Meal Plan

DAY	BREAKFAST	MAIN DISH	SIDE	DESSERT
1	Pumpkin Spice Smoothie	Curry Spiced Lentil Burgers	Jackfruit Carnitas	Mint Chocolate Chip Sorbet
2	Mint Chocolate Smoothie	Cajun Burgers	Aloo Gobi	Minty Fruit Salad
3	Pineapple Breeze Smoothie	Maple Dijon Burgers	Baked Beans	Cherry-Vanilla Rice Pudding
4	Super Green Smoothie	Grilled AHLT	Aloo Gobi	Mint Chocolate Chip Sorbet
5	Pumpkin Spice Smoothie	Mediterranean Hummus Pizza	Aloo Gobi	Cherry-Vanilla Rice Pudding
6	Super Green Smoothie	Curry Spiced Lentil Burgers	Jambalaya	Minty Fruit Salad

7	Mint Chocolate Smoothie	Maple Dijon Burgers	Jackfruit Carnitas	Minty Fruit Salad
8	Pumpkin Spice Smoothie	Cajun Burgers	Baked Beans	Banana Chocolate Cupcakes
9	Mint Chocolate Smoothie	Grilled AHLT	Aloo Gobi	Minty Fruit Salad
10	Pineapple Breeze Smoothie	Maple Dijon Burgers	Brussels Sprouts Curry	Mint Chocolate Chip Sorbet
11	Super Green Smoothie	Black Bean Pizza	Aloo Gobi	Cherry-Vanilla Rice Pudding
12	Pumpkin Spice Smoothie	Mediterranean Hummus Pizza	Baked Beans	Banana Chocolate Cupcakes
13	Pumpkin Spice Smoothie	Curry Spiced Lentil Burgers	Jackfruit Carnitas	Minty Fruit Salad
14	Mint Chocolate Smoothie	Cajun Burgers	Jambalaya	Minty Fruit Salad

15	Mint Chocolate Smoothie	Maple Dijon Burgers	Aloo Gobi	Banana Chocolate Cupcakes
16	Pineapple Breeze Smoothie	Curry Spiced Lentil Burgers	Aloo Gobi	Minty Fruit Salad
17	Pumpkin Spice Smoothie	Mediterranean Hummus Pizza	Brussels Sprouts Curry	Mint Chocolate Chip Sorbet
18	Super Green Smoothie	Grilled AHLT	Jackfruit Carnitas	Peach-Mango Crumble
19	Super Green Smoothie	Black Bean Pizza	Jambalaya	Minty Fruit Salad
20	Pumpkin Spice Smoothie	Cajun Burgers	Brussels Sprouts Curry	Banana Chocolate Cupcakes
21	Pineapple Breeze Smoothie	Curry Spiced Lentil Burgers	Baked Beans	Cherry-Vanilla Rice Pudding
22	Mint Chocolate Smoothie	Mediterranean Hummus Pizza	Aloo Gobi	Minty Fruit Salad
23	Super Green Smoothie	Grilled AHLT	Aloo Gobi	Banana Chocolate Cupcakes

24	Pumpkin Spice Smoothie	Cajun Burgers	Jambalaya	Mint Chocolate Chip Sorbet
25	Pineapple Breeze Smoothie	Maple Dijon Burgers	Jackfruit Carnitas	Cherry-Vanilla Rice Pudding
26	Pumpkin Spice Smoothie	Curry Spiced Lentil Burgers	Brussels Sprouts Curry	Minty Fruit Salad
27	Super Green Smoothie	Black Bean Pizza	Aloo Gobi	Cherry-Vanilla Rice Pudding
28	Mint Chocolate Smoothie	Cajun Burgers	Jackfruit Carnitas	Banana Chocolate Cupcakes
29	Pumpkin Spice Smoothie	Curry Spiced Lentil Burgers	Baked Beans	Mango Coconut Cream Pie
30	Pineapple Breeze Smoothie	Grilled AHLT	Aloo Gobi	Minty Fruit Salad

Conclusion

As an athlete, it may sound like the vegan diet may not provide you the right nutrition. Rest assured; you can very well debunk that myth.

Over the course of the book, I've given you a bunch of tasty and easy to make recipes that will surely provide you fair share of carbohydrates and protein. Keep in mind that being meat-free athlete isn't simple, this is barely a reason to quit!

One of the utmost benefits of shifting into vegan is the improved level of health that you will undergo and this will show well beyond on your physique. In addition to this, the strong combination of healthy plant-based protein! The vegan diet is famous for its health benefits and especially for weight loss. Many people have made a vegan diet to lose weight and have succeeded.

Lose weight, enjoy more energy, and feel good by making a difference in vegetarianism. But before starting a vegan diet, you may be looking for a healthy and healthy diet to lose weight, and there are some things you should understand.

Most people make the mistake of giving the word 'diet' a negative connotation. It is for this reason that most of them are unable to stick to a diet when they want to switch to a different lifestyle. It is important that you do not do that. Tell yourself that you are switching to a healthier lifestyle that has numerous benefits. Remember that it is okay to give yourself one cheat meal. You can consume this meal on those days when you have cravings. You should remember to never make a habit out of it. Once you begin to lead a vegan lifestyle fully, you will no longer have any meat cravings.

Those who switch to a vegan diet get immediate benefits on their strength and note a better and faster muscle development. For an athlete also should not be underestimated the advantage of boosting the immune system, since it allows him to get sick less frequently and therefore, he can focus better on training.

Furthermore, in vegan nutrition there are no foods that are in fact pro-inflammatory, such as meat and dairy products, rich in cholesterol and saturated fats.

However, we should not make the mistake of believing that it suffices to be vegan so that everything goes well. Like any kind of nutrition, we need to make sure to incorporate a good variety of nutrient-rich food sources.

It is a good idea to structure a good personalized plan of weekly meals in order to be sure of assimilating everything the body needs. It is also good to feed several times a day and tossing away the famous rule of "three meals a day." High-end athletes eat up to 8-9 times a day, following their personalized nutritional program.

To be well prepared, the key is to have an unmistakable objective for the occasion, stick to individual plans and readiness procedures, remain at the time, and limit the effect of interruptions. Staying positive and hopeful, even despite misfortune, and overseeing feelings every day are extra tips that can have a major effect once rivalry shows up. For the groups who are set up for the experience, rivalries give energizing chances to exhibit capacities and are significant learning open doors for youthful athletes.

Now that you have learned the benefits of switching to a vegan lifestyle, and understand that there are ample plant-based or nut-based proteins that can help you provide your body with the necessary protein and other nutrients, it is time for you to get started with the recipes.